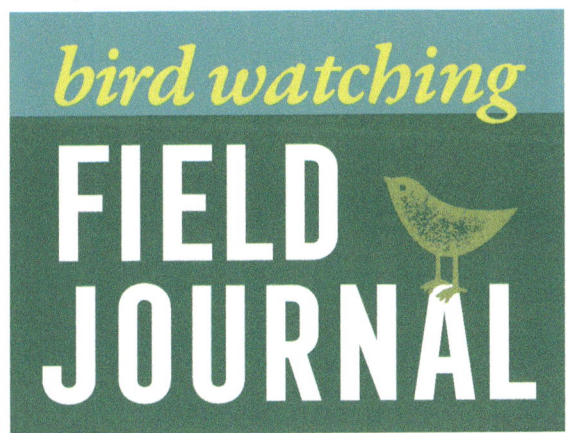

bird watching FIELD JOURNAL

LOG, SKETCHBOOK, AND LIFE LIST

Kristine Rivers

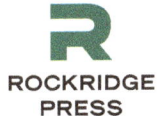

ROCKRIDGE PRESS

Copyright © 2022 by Rockridge Press, Oakland, California

No part of this publication may be reproduced, stored in a retrieval system, or transmitted in any form or by any means, electronic, mechanical, photocopying, recording, scanning, or otherwise, except as permitted under Sections 107 or 108 of the 1976 United States Copyright Act, without the prior written permission of the Publisher. Requests to the Publisher for permission should be addressed to the Permissions Department, Rockridge Press, 1955 Broadway, Suite 400, Oakland, CA 94612.

Limit of Liability/Disclaimer of Warranty: The Publisher and the author make no representations or warranties with respect to the accuracy or completeness of the contents of this work and specifically disclaim all warranties, including without limitation warranties of fitness for a particular purpose. No warranty may be created or extended by sales or promotional materials. The advice and strategies contained herein may not be suitable for every situation. This work is sold with the understanding that the Publisher is not engaged in rendering medical, legal, or other professional advice or services. If professional assistance is required, the services of a competent professional person should be sought. Neither the Publisher nor the author shall be liable for damages arising herefrom. The fact that an individual, organization, or website is referred to in this work as a citation and/or potential source of further information does not mean that the author or the Publisher endorses the information the individual, organization, or website may provide or recommendations they/it may make. Further, readers should be aware that websites listed in this work may have changed or disappeared between when this work was written and when it is read. For general information on our other products and services or to obtain technical support, please contact our Customer Care Department within the United States at (866) 744-2665, or outside the United States at (510) 253-0500.

Rockridge Press publishes its books in a variety of electronic and print formats. Some content that appears in print may not be available in electronic books, and vice versa.

TRADEMARKS: Rockridge Press and the Rockridge Press logo are trademarks or registered trademarks of Callisto Media Inc. and/or its affiliates, in the United States and other countries, and may not be used without written permission. All other trademarks are the property of their respective owners. Rockridge Press is not associated with any product or vendor mentioned in this book.

Interior and Cover Designer: Jami Spittler
Art Producer: Sue Bischofberger
Editor: Anne Goldberg
Production Editor: Ashley Polikoff

Photography used under license from shutterstock.com and iStockphoto.com.
Author photo courtesy of LA Capturing Moments Photography.
Illustration used under license from shutterstock.com.

ISBN: 978-1-638-78571-2
R0

Printed in Canada

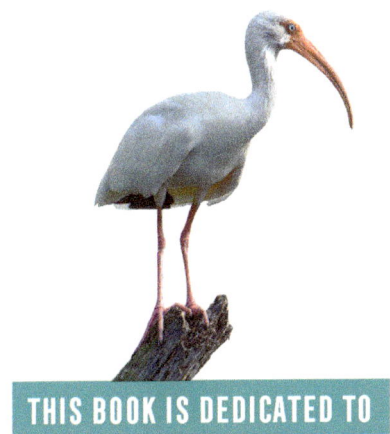

THIS BOOK IS DEDICATED TO

my son, Julian, and my husband, Bobby,
who can probably recite
my birding tips in their sleep!

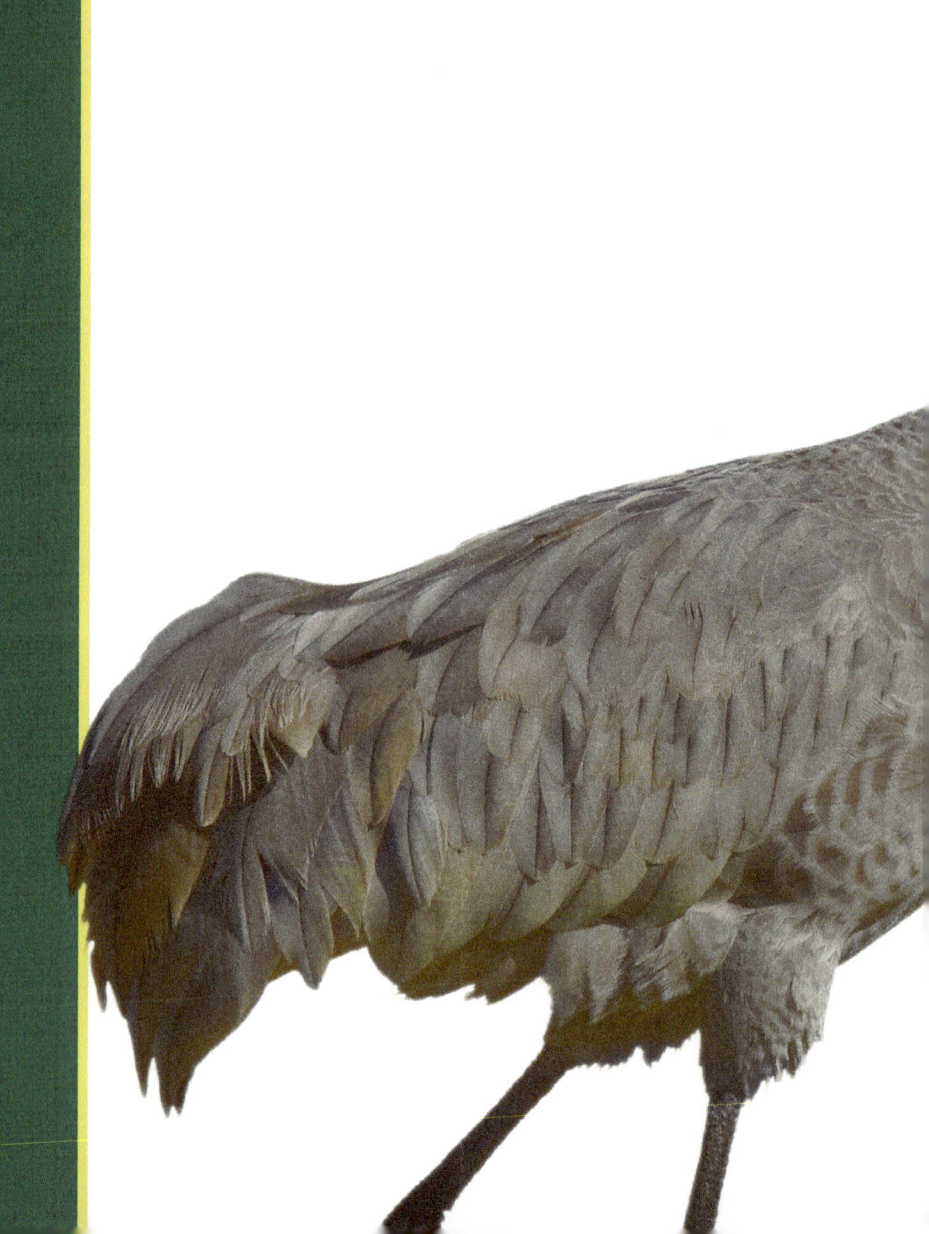

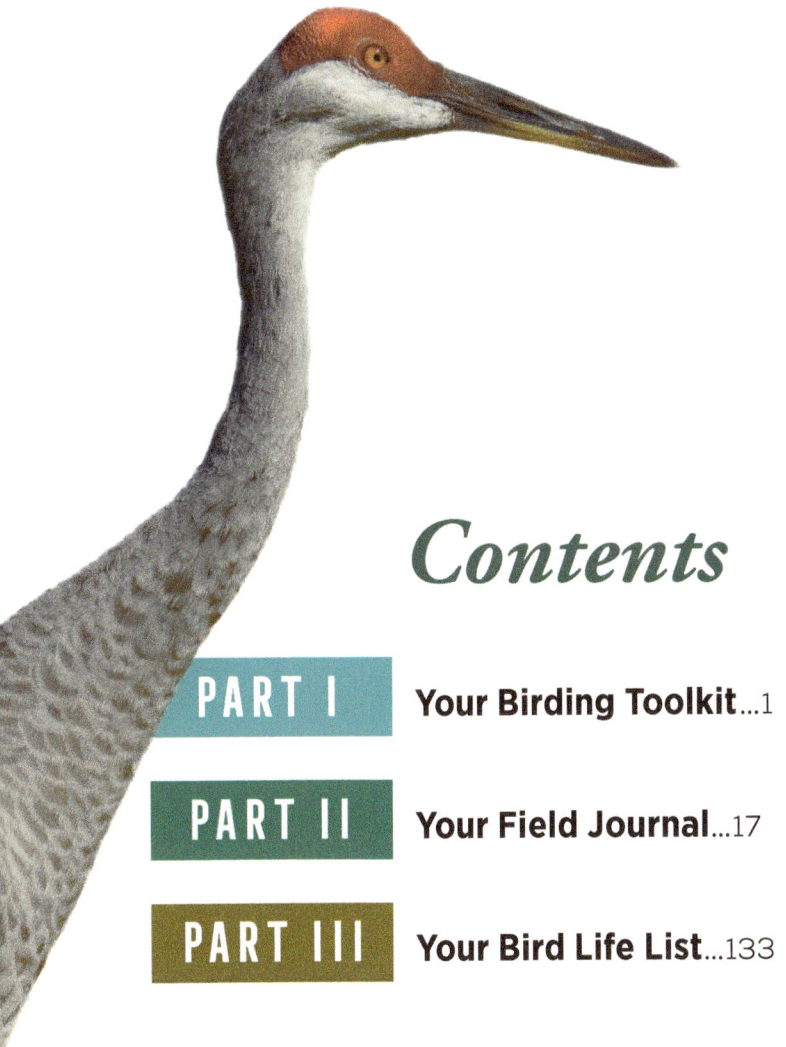

Contents

PART I   **Your Birding Toolkit**...1

PART II   **Your Field Journal**...17

PART III   **Your Bird Life List**...133

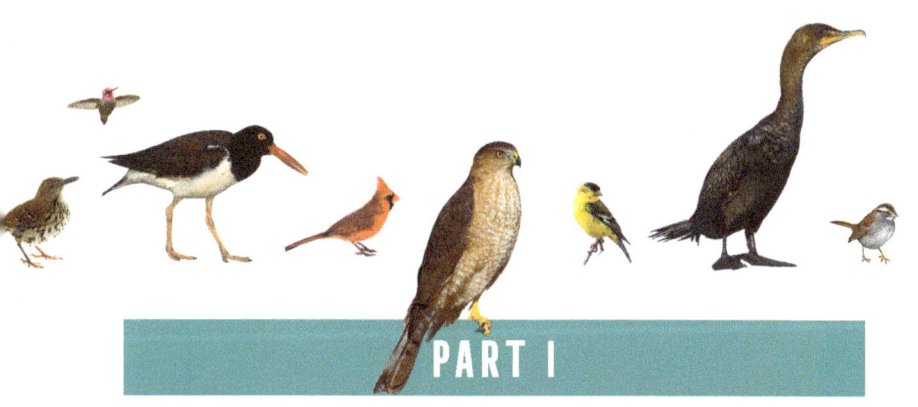

PART I

YOUR BIRDING TOOLKIT

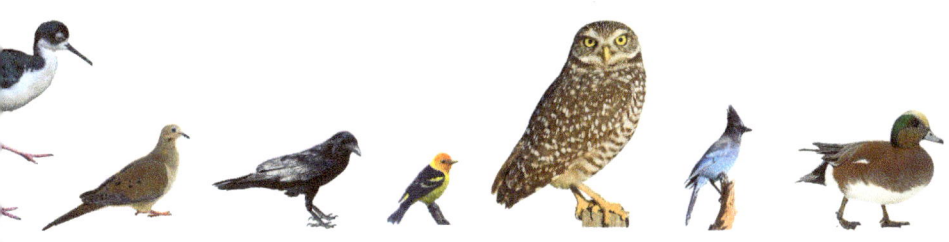

FIELD TIPS

Welcome to the world of birding! People from all different backgrounds enjoy watching birds, whether in their own yard, in local parks, or while traveling. It's a great activity for both physical and mental health, fun for all ages, and provides continuous learning opportunities. It's also reasonably inexpensive: All you need are a good pair of binoculars and a field guide to get started!

Here are a few tips to help you prepare for your adventures:

STAY SAFE. Many areas that are great for birding are also remote. Explore with a birding buddy, and make sure someone knows where you're going. Carry your cell phone with you and keep it charged. Additionally, stay on established trails.

DRESS APPROPRIATELY. Wearing muted earth tones will help you blend into your surroundings, whereas white or brightly colored clothing may scare birds away. Wear footwear that will protect your feet, such as walking shoes or hiking boots. Bring a hat or visor to shade your face from the sun, if needed.

PREPARE FOR CHANGES IN THE WEATHER. Check the weather in advance so you know what to expect. Wear layers so you can adjust your clothing throughout the day to stay comfortable. Bring extra clothing with you.

PROTECT YOUR SKIN. Long pants will protect your legs from insect bites, scratches, poison ivy, poison oak, and other irritants. In an area with chiggers, tuck your pant legs into your socks to avoid getting bitten. Wear insect repellant and sunscreen when needed.

PACK A BAG. Create a birding bag from a waterproof backpack or similar bag so you'll always be ready to explore. Your field guide, journal, and writing tools should be placed in the top or sides of the bag, so you can pull them out quickly. Pack your sunscreen, bug spray, and a small first aid kit in a different pocket or at the bottom of the bag. Don't forget snacks for an energy boost, and bottled water to stay hydrated.

KNOW YOUR SURROUNDINGS. Many parks and wildlife refuges provide maps and other detailed information both online and in print form. Ask for birding checklists, which tell you what species can be seen in different seasons and how common they are. Bring along trail maps when hiking, even in familiar locations.

FOLLOW BIRDING ETIQUETTE. Never trespass on private property. Approach other birders and wildlife enthusiasts quietly to avoid scaring animals they are viewing. Use recorded bird calls only as a reference, not to attract birds, as they can disturb threatened, endangered, or nesting species within their territories. Never deliberately disturb or flush birds. Be sure to leave the habitat as you found it.

IDENTIFYING YOUR BIRD

To effectively identify a bird, consider it within its overall surroundings in addition to how it looks. Browse your field guide or app *before* going birding. Observe as much as you can about the bird before opening your field guide. Take notes, make sketches, or capture a few quick photographs to reference later, if needed.

Remember, identification is simply a process of elimination. Here are some factors that will help you narrow down your choices:

GROUP

Having a general idea of a bird's family will help you find it more easily in your field guide. Start by deciding if you're observing a *land bird* or *water bird*.

LAND BIRDS: Includes fowl-like birds that live on the ground (similar to grouse or quail), tree-dwellers (songbirds, woodpeckers, hummingbirds, etc.), and raptors (like hawks, eagles, and owls).

WATER BIRDS: Includes swimmers (ducks and duck-like birds), aerialists (gulls and gull-like birds), long-legged waders (like herons and cranes), and smaller waders (such as sandpipers or plovers).

SIZE

Now estimate the overall *size* of your bird to help sort through potential species.

COMPARE THE SIZE TO A KNOWN SPECIES. If your mystery bird is obviously smaller than the Northern Mockingbirds you see frequently, and your guide says that mockingbirds are around nine inches in length, you can automatically eliminate all potential species larger than that.

COMPARE THE SIZE TO A MEASURABLE OBJECT. You can also compare your bird's size with something you can measure, such as your shoe or backpack. If you estimate your mystery bird to be about the same size as your 15-inch backpack, you can automatically eliminate potential species smaller than that.

SHAPE

Noting the *shape* or silhouette created by your bird's entire body will help you determine its family group (songbird, hummingbird, duck, hawk, etc.). In addition to its overall silhouette, carefully observe the shape of each part of your bird.

HEAD: Is the top of its head *flat* like a wren, *round* like a chickadee, *peaked* like a flycatcher, or *crested* like a cardinal?

BODY: Is the body *slender* or *plump*?

BEAK: Is the bill *long* or *short*? *Straight* or *curved*? Is it *fine and tweezer-shaped* for catching insects? *Short and sturdy* for cracking seeds? *Dagger-shaped* for catching fish? *Hooked at the tip* for tearing prey apart? *Chisel-shaped* for finding insects under tree bark? *Thin and tubular* for drinking nectar?

WINGS: In flight, are the wingtips *pointed* or *rounded*? Are the wings *straight* like an eagle or *bent at the wrist* like a tern? When folded, do the wings *extend past the tail* or are they *shorter than the tail*?

TAIL: Is the tail *long* or *short* compared to the bird's body? Is the end of the tail *squared*, *rounded*, *pointed*, slightly *notched*, or deeply *forked*?

LEGS: Are its legs *long* like a heron or *short* like a tern?

FIELD MARKS

A bird's *field marks*—distinctive stripes, spots, colors, and patterns—can narrow identification down further to species.

HEAD: Look for patches of color on the *crown*, *cheek*, and *throat*. Are there *crown stripes* or lines on top of the head? Does it have an *eyebrow* line above the eye, *eyeline* going through the eye, or *whisker line* below the eye? If it has a colored *eye-ring* encircling the eye, is it full or broken? Subtle or bold? Are the eye-rings connected over the beak to form *spectacles*? Is there a colored *lore spot* between the eye and beak? Does it look like it's wearing a *mask* or *hood*? Is the throat *plain* or *streaked*?

BODY: Is the *back* a distinct color? Is there a patch of color on the *rump* above the tail? Or colored *undertail covert* feathers beneath the tail? Are the *breast* and *belly* unmarked? Or *spotted*, *streaked* with up-and-down stripes, or *barred* with side-to-side stripes? Does it look like it's wearing a *bib*? Do you see any color on the *flanks*, just under the wings?

WINGS: When the wings are folded, do you see any *wing bars*, or lines of contrasting color? If so, how many? Are they subtle or bold? When the wings are extended in flight, are there any large *patches* (blocks of color) or *barring*? Is there a different color along the *leading* or *trailing edges* of the wings?

TAIL: Is the *tail* a distinct color? Are there *white tips* at the end, *white patches* on the corners, or *white outer tail feathers*? Is there *barring*? If so, is the barring *thin* or *wide*? Is there a *terminal band* of a different color on the end of the tail?

COLOR

Although the main colors of a bird may be helpful in identification, color itself isn't the most important feature. For example, a "green bird" could describe anything from a parakeet to a heron. Pay attention to *where* color appears on the body as well as the *shade* of that color. For example, a male Northern Cardinal has a bright red head and body, an American Robin has a rusty red breast, and a male Downy Woodpecker has a tiny red patch on the back of its crown. General impressions can also be helpful, such as noticing that a bird is dark above and light below while in flight.

PLUMAGE

The overall colors and patterns, or *plumages*, of birds include all visible body parts—feathers, eyes, beaks, facial skin, legs, and feet. Plumage varies based on age and gender of the bird and changes in appearance throughout the year. Birds also *molt*, or replace their feathers, further altering their appearance. This means that plumages vary from one species to another and within the same species as well.

- Most field guides distinguish between *non-breeding* or *basic plumage* (worn during fall/winter) and *breeding* or *alternate plumage* (worn briefly during spring/summer). Species that look the same year-round are always in basic plumage.

- Adult males often vary in plumage from adult females. In species where genders have similar coloration, females are often larger.

🐦 Immature birds vary in plumage from adults because young birds need downy, well-camouflaged feathers for protection, whereas adults need feathers that will support flight and attract mates. Large species such as the Bald Eagle take several years to transition, looking distinctly different from year to year.

🐦 Regional variations sometimes occur, in which the same species has different plumage coloration depending on where it occurs. For instance, the Northern Flicker has two varieties: Red-shafted (western birds with red feathers in wings and tail) and Yellow-shafted (eastern birds with yellow feathers in wings and tail).

🐦 Some species also have distinct *color morphs* or forms exhibited by adults. This is different from a *phase*, in which an individual bird's color changes over time.

Suffice it to say these plumage variations can make identification difficult! Just remember to consider season and location in addition to age and gender when identifying a bird. Be sure to look at all the illustrations or photos provided for each species in your field guide; those with plainer plumage are easy to overlook, but just as important as those with colorful plumage.

BEHAVIOR

Birds have adapted their behaviors over time to take advantage of their environments and avoid direct competition with other species. Behavioral clues will narrow possibilities during identification.

PERCHED BIRD: Is it *out in the open* or *hiding in vegetation*? Does its body posture look *horizontal* like a nighthawk or *vertical* like a bluebird? Does it hold its tail *up* like a wren or *down* like a flycatcher? Is it resting with *head tucked under its wing* or *standing on one leg* like a sandpiper?

FLYING BIRD: Is it *flying solo* or *in a flock*? Does it *soar* like an eagle, *flap its wings* like a crow, or *hover in the air* like a hummingbird? Does it have *fast* or *slow wingbeats*? Does it fly *straight through the air* or *swoop up and down*?

CLIMBING BIRD: Is it *making short upward jumps* like a woodpecker? Does it look like it's *climbing a spiral staircase* like a creeper? Or is it *going down the tree headfirst* like a nuthatch?

SWIMMING BIRD: Does it sit *high in the water* like a duck or *low in the water* like a cormorant? Does it forage with *just its head underwater* or *dive underwater completely*?

WADING BIRD: Is it *wading in shallow water* like a Sanderling or *wading belly deep* like a dowitcher? Is it *foraging by sight* (watching for prey or picking items from the sand's surface)? Or is it *foraging by feel* (sweeping its beak through the water or probing it deep into mud)?

EATING BIRD: Is it foraging for plant-based food (*eating seeds* from the ground, *picking berries* from the treetops, or *drinking nectar* from flowers)? Or is it searching for animal-based food (*chasing insects*, *catching fish*, or *hunting mammals*)? Or is it eating a *combination of foods*, like a robin that eats both worms and berries?

OTHER BEHAVIORS: Watch for repetitive movements such as the *head bob* of a yellowlegs or the *tail pump* of a kestrel. Notice whether your bird is interacting with other birds. When a bird is *preening* or *bathing*, look for plumage details.

VOICE

You don't need to be able to identify birdsongs to be a good birder. Remember, birds sing mostly during breeding season, in late spring and early summer. They make many other noises throughout the year, such as chips, warning calls, hammering, and rustling—just follow the sound until you find the bird making it. You will find more birds by listening carefully, especially in habitats such as woodlands and marshes where birds take cover for protection.

HABITAT

Habitats must provide the resources birds need for survival: food, water, space, and shelter. Though birds live in nearly every type of environment, each species lives in habitats that meet their own specific needs. Understanding the species associated with each habitat will help you narrow down identification possibilities.

The four basic habitat types are:

AQUATIC: Habitat with water, including areas covered with water all or some of the time. Swimmers, aerialists, and waders can be found here. Understanding which species prefer *saltwater*, *freshwater*, or *brackish water* (a mixture of the two) can aid in identification. For example, most egrets live in both salt- and freshwater habitats; however, the Reddish Egret is a saltwater specialist, so you won't usually find it in a freshwater habitat.

WOODLAND: Habitat with many mature trees and plants, that is more open than a forest. Tree-dwellers and birds of prey can be found here. Determining the *kinds of trees* (deciduous hardwood, coniferous/pine, mixed, etc.) and the *density of the understory* can help you decide between similar species. For instance, whereas Downy Woodpeckers may be found in deciduous or mixed woodlands, including those in urban areas, Red-cockaded Woodpeckers will be found only in mature stands of pine trees with minimal understory.

GRASSLAND: Wide-open habitat where mostly grasses and flowers grow. Ground-dwellers and birds of prey can be found here. Understanding which species prefer vegetation that is *tall and dense* or *managed* (mowed, etc.) will aid in identification. For example, Henslow's Sparrows may be seen in pastures with tall grass, but Grasshopper Sparrows avoid pastures that are too overgrown.

SCRUB-SHRUB: Habitat sparsely covered with low, woody vegetation such as bushes and young trees. Some tree-dwellers can be found here. Understanding which species prefer *scraggly habitats without mature trees* can help with identification. Although the Dusky Flycatcher can be seen in brushy areas and arid scrub, the similar-looking Hammond's Flycatcher will be found only in mature, old-growth forests.

RANGE

Birders use range (distribution) maps to find out *where* a species is most likely to occur because different birds "match" different habitats. Once you have identification narrowed down to one or two possibilities, checking the range of each species can be an easy way to decide between them. For example, although the Carolina Chickadee and Black-capped Chickadee look nearly identical, their ranges are very different.

SEASON

Range maps also indicate *when* a species is most likely to occur in any given area. Although some birds are *year-round* residents, most *migrate* seasonally from one location to another. For that reason, the possible species you might encounter in your area vary depending on the season. Phenomena known as *groundings* or *fallouts* occur during spring and fall migrations when dramatic weather changes, such as strong winds and rain, can force thousands of migrating birds to the ground.

Birds may be much easier to find during *breeding season* in late spring and early summer, when they can be heard vocalizing and seen defending their territories. A greater diversity of species may be seen during *nonbreeding season* in fall and winter, when they may be more willing to share territories with one another.

HOW TO USE THIS JOURNAL

Keeping a birding journal is a great way to help you remember details about birds you see in the field. It enables you to record information quickly, during or just after a sighting, while your impressions and observations are fresh. Be sure to make notes *before* consulting any reference materials for help with identification. It's easy to get confused about what you actually saw once you start looking through all the pictures in your field guide. It can also be difficult to research identification of a bird while actively watching it, so your notes will be a valuable reference when you have a better opportunity to do so. In the case of an unusual or rare sighting, contemporaneous notes and sketches are useful to experts to confirm species identification.

Your birding journal isn't just for documenting species that are new to you, however; making notes and sketching key features will help sharpen your *observation* skills as well as your identification skills. With practice, you will train your eyes and brain to automatically focus on details such as the shape of the beak, the length of the tail, flight pattern, etc. You may also want to add notes to an entry after the fact, such as information you discovered that helped with identification or things to look for if you see the bird again. Recording sentimental memories of birding excursions and exciting sightings will make it fun to review or share with others later. Be creative—it's your journal!

DATE & TIME

Note the date and time you first spotted your bird. You can also include the season (spring, summer, fall, winter). This helps you learn whether the bird is a resident or a migrant in your area and if there are certain times of day it is usually seen.

SPECIES NAME

If you know the species, add the common name and scientific name of your bird. If you're not sure, you can use your journal notes to identify what you saw, and then add the names later. Remember, it's okay not to be able to identify a bird right away!
    Example:
COMMON NAME: Red-tailed Hawk
SCIENTIFIC NAME: *Buteo jamaicensis*

LOCATION

Note general information about where you saw the bird, such as city and state and the name of park or refuge, private property, etc. If accuracy is needed (to provide documentation of a rare species, for example) you can use GPS to record exact coordinates. It's also helpful to include specific details about where you saw your bird, such as in a tree, flying overhead, or on the ground. Add notes about habitat, nearby water or food sources, types of trees or plants, or other birds in the area.

WEATHER

Add the temperature if you know it; if not, note how the weather feels: warm, hot, cool, or cold. You can also note the wind—gusty, slight breeze, still—and other weather conditions that might affect your ability to see the bird, like rain, mist, fog, or snow. Be sure to note visibility: sunny and clear, partly cloudy, and overcast are all good descriptions.

FIELD NOTES

This is where you get to be really descriptive about your bird! First, make notes about its appearance:

- How big is your bird?
- What is the shape of its overall body? Does its body look plump or slender?

- What are the shapes of its individual body parts: the beak, top of its head, wings, tail, or legs?
- What are the main colors of its overall plumage? What about the colors of specific body parts, like the eyes, beak, legs, and feet?
- Do you see any obvious field marks on the bird's head, body, wings, or tail? Do you see patterns such as streaking, barring, or spotting on its feathers?
- Do you notice any unusual features, such as missing feathers?

Now add notes about the bird's behavior or actions:

- What is your bird doing—resting, foraging, preening, bathing, flying, swimming?
- How is your bird moving? Is it walking or hopping on the ground? Soaring or flapping its wings in flight? Climbing a tree trunk or jumping between branches? Wading or swimming in water?
- Is your bird eating anything? How is it gathering its food?
- Is it interacting with other birds? If so, how?
- Is it singing or making any other noises?

THE SKETCH PAD

Use this area to draw quick sketches of your bird while in the field. Add things that might help you identify it later, such as its shape, body parts (beak, field marks, feet), or movement (flying back and forth, wagging its tail). Remember, your sketches don't have to be perfect! Just try to capture your overall impression of the bird and any features that draw your attention during observation.

DATE & TIME: DECEMBER 18, 2021, 8:30 A.M.

SPECIES NAME: RED-TAILED HAWK (BUTEO JAMAICENSIS)

LOCATION: BRAZOS BEND STATE PARK, NEEDVILLE, TX

WEATHER: 54 DEGREES, SUNNY AND CLEAR, CHILLY BUT TEMPS RISING

SIZE & SHAPE: LARGE RAPTOR WITH FANNED TAIL

BEAK SHAPE: NOT VISIBLE FROM UNDERNEATH

WING SHAPE: BROAD WINGS, ROUNDED ON THE ENDS, WITH FINGERLIKE FEATHERS

COLOR/PLUMAGE: LIGHT-COLORED OR WHITE UNDERNEATH AND BROWN ON HEAD AND BACK

FIELD MARKS: BROWN STREAKING IN A BAND ACROSS WHITE BELLY, DARK TRAILING EDGES ON THE WINGS, RUSTY TAIL

FIELD NOTES: BIRD IDENTIFIED BY FELLOW BIRDERS DURING CHRISTMAS BIRD COUNT. IT WAS SOARING EFFORTLESSLY IN BROAD CIRCLES ABOVE US, RIDING THE THERMALS WITHOUT FLAPPING. THE RUSTY TAIL CONTRASTED WITH THE DARKER BACK.

SKETCH PAD

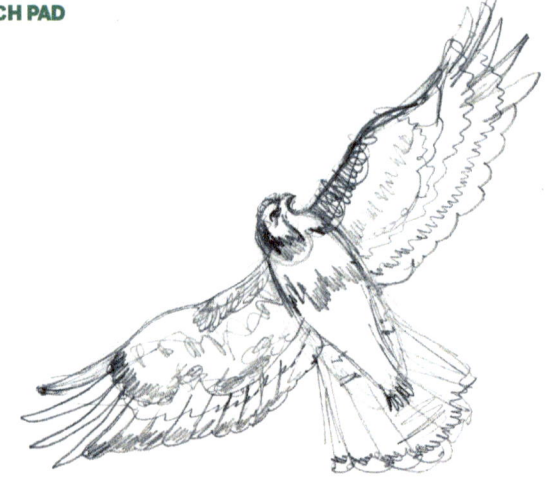

HOW TO COMPLETE YOUR LIFE LIST

Many birders keep a "life list" to record all the bird species they have ever seen. You can use the following pages to start your list. Begin by adding common species you know you have already seen, even if you don't know the exact date—just note the year or "unsure" on those entries. When you see a species that is new to you, record the date, species name, and location on your list. This will help you remember when and where you first saw each species. It will also keep track of the total number of species you have seen since you first started birding. Your list will increase naturally as you spend more time birding and become better at identification. You also may enjoy purposely seeking out new species by exploring in your own area and by visiting birding hot spots. Join birding groups online or sign up for rare bird alerts to learn about any unusual species when they occur in your area. Some people are quite competitive about it!

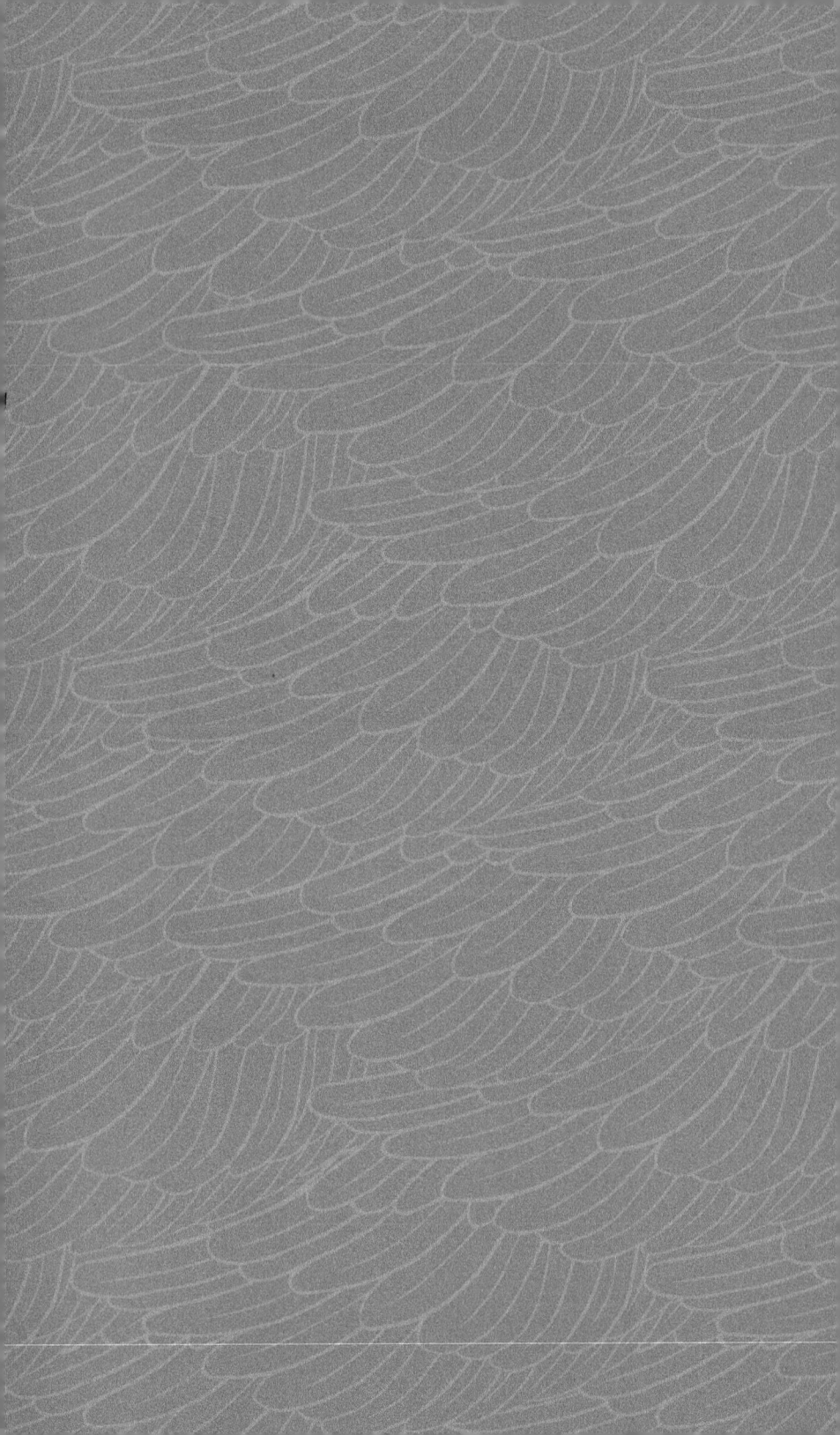

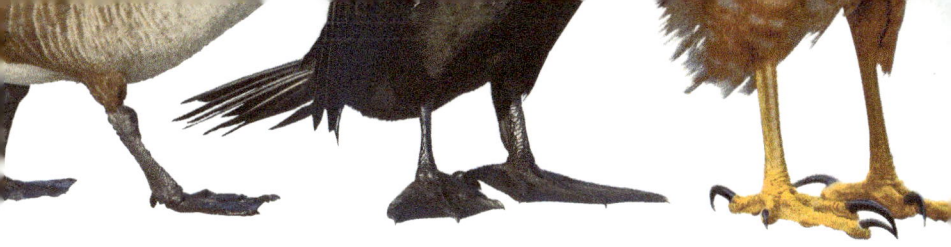

PART II

YOUR FIELD JOURNAL

Now you're ready to fill the journal pages in this section with observations from your birding adventures! Each page includes suggestions of what to record, with room for additional notes and sketches so you can make each entry your own. Let your curiosity lead you and have fun capturing your memories here.

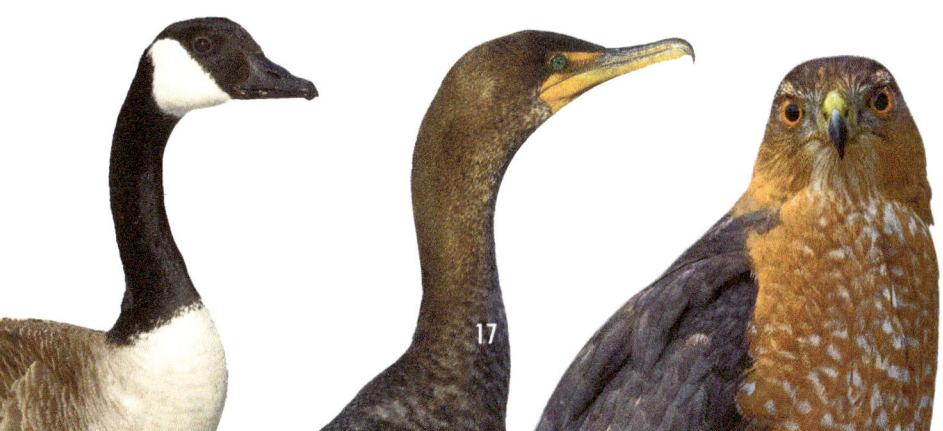

DATE & TIME: _____

SPECIES NAME: _____

LOCATION: _____

WEATHER: _____

SIZE & SHAPE: _____

BEAK SHAPE: _____

WING SHAPE: _____

_____

COLOR/PLUMAGE: _____

FIELD MARKS: _____

_____

FIELD NOTES: _____

_____

_____

_____

SKETCH PAD

DATE & TIME: _____

SPECIES NAME: _____

LOCATION: _____

WEATHER: _____

SIZE & SHAPE: _____

BEAK SHAPE: _____

WING SHAPE: _____

_____

COLOR/PLUMAGE: _____

FIELD MARKS: _____

_____

FIELD NOTES: _____

_____

_____

_____

SKETCH PAD

DATE & TIME: _____

SPECIES NAME: _____

LOCATION: _____

WEATHER: _____

SIZE & SHAPE: _____

BEAK SHAPE: _____

WING SHAPE: _____

_____

COLOR/PLUMAGE: _____

FIELD MARKS: _____

_____

FIELD NOTES: _____

_____

_____

_____

SKETCH PAD

DATE & TIME: _____

SPECIES NAME: _____

LOCATION: _____

WEATHER: _____

SIZE & SHAPE: _____

BEAK SHAPE: _____

WING SHAPE: _____

_____

COLOR/PLUMAGE: _____

FIELD MARKS: _____

_____

FIELD NOTES: _____

_____

_____

_____

SKETCH PAD

DATE & TIME: _____

SPECIES NAME: _____

LOCATION: _____

WEATHER: _____

SIZE & SHAPE: _____

BEAK SHAPE: _____

WING SHAPE: _____

_____

COLOR/PLUMAGE: _____

FIELD MARKS: _____

_____

FIELD NOTES: _____

_____

_____

_____

SKETCH PAD

DATE & TIME: _____

SPECIES NAME: _____

LOCATION: _____

WEATHER: _____

SIZE & SHAPE: _____

BEAK SHAPE: _____

WING SHAPE: _____

_____

COLOR/PLUMAGE: _____

FIELD MARKS: _____

_____

FIELD NOTES: _____

_____

_____

_____

SKETCH PAD

DATE & TIME: _____

SPECIES NAME: _____

LOCATION: _____

WEATHER: _____

SIZE & SHAPE: _____

BEAK SHAPE: _____

WING SHAPE: _____

_____

COLOR/PLUMAGE: _____

FIELD MARKS: _____

_____

FIELD NOTES: _____

_____

_____

_____

SKETCH PAD

DATE & TIME: _____

SPECIES NAME: _____

LOCATION: _____

WEATHER: _____

SIZE & SHAPE: _____

BEAK SHAPE: _____

WING SHAPE: _____

_____

COLOR/PLUMAGE: _____

FIELD MARKS: _____

_____

FIELD NOTES: _____

_____

_____

_____

SKETCH PAD

DATE & TIME: _____

SPECIES NAME: _____

LOCATION: _____

WEATHER: _____

SIZE & SHAPE: _____

BEAK SHAPE: _____

WING SHAPE: _____

_____

COLOR/PLUMAGE: _____

FIELD MARKS: _____

_____

FIELD NOTES: _____

_____

_____

_____

SKETCH PAD

DATE & TIME: _____

SPECIES NAME: _____

LOCATION: _____

WEATHER: _____

SIZE & SHAPE: _____

BEAK SHAPE: _____

WING SHAPE: _____

_____

COLOR/PLUMAGE: _____

FIELD MARKS: _____

_____

FIELD NOTES: _____

_____

_____

_____

SKETCH PAD

DATE & TIME: _____

SPECIES NAME: _____

LOCATION: _____

WEATHER: _____

SIZE & SHAPE: _____

BEAK SHAPE: _____

WING SHAPE: _____

_____

COLOR/PLUMAGE: _____

FIELD MARKS: _____

_____

FIELD NOTES: _____

_____

_____

_____

SKETCH PAD

DATE & TIME: _____

SPECIES NAME: _____

LOCATION: _____

WEATHER: _____

SIZE & SHAPE: _____

BEAK SHAPE: _____

WING SHAPE: _____

_____

COLOR/PLUMAGE: _____

FIELD MARKS: _____

_____

FIELD NOTES: _____

_____

_____

_____

SKETCH PAD

DATE & TIME: _____

SPECIES NAME: _____

LOCATION: _____

WEATHER: _____

SIZE & SHAPE: _____

BEAK SHAPE: _____

WING SHAPE: _____

_____

COLOR/PLUMAGE: _____

FIELD MARKS: _____

_____

FIELD NOTES: _____

_____

_____

_____

SKETCH PAD

DATE & TIME: _____

SPECIES NAME: _____

LOCATION: _____

WEATHER: _____

SIZE & SHAPE: _____

BEAK SHAPE: _____

WING SHAPE: _____

_____

COLOR/PLUMAGE: _____

FIELD MARKS: _____

_____

FIELD NOTES: _____

_____

_____

_____

SKETCH PAD

DATE & TIME: _____

SPECIES NAME: _____

LOCATION: _____

WEATHER: _____

SIZE & SHAPE: _____

BEAK SHAPE: _____

WING SHAPE: _____

_____

COLOR/PLUMAGE: _____

FIELD MARKS: _____

_____

FIELD NOTES: _____

_____

_____

_____

SKETCH PAD

DATE & TIME: _____

SPECIES NAME: _____

LOCATION: _____

WEATHER: _____

SIZE & SHAPE: _____

BEAK SHAPE: _____

WING SHAPE: _____

_____

COLOR/PLUMAGE: _____

FIELD MARKS: _____

_____

FIELD NOTES: _____

_____

_____

_____

SKETCH PAD

DATE & TIME: _____

SPECIES NAME: _____

LOCATION: _____

WEATHER: _____

SIZE & SHAPE: _____

BEAK SHAPE: _____

WING SHAPE: _____

_____

COLOR/PLUMAGE: _____

FIELD MARKS: _____

_____

FIELD NOTES: _____

_____

_____

_____

SKETCH PAD

DATE & TIME: _____

SPECIES NAME: _____

LOCATION: _____

WEATHER: _____

SIZE & SHAPE: _____

BEAK SHAPE: _____

WING SHAPE: _____

_____

COLOR/PLUMAGE: _____

FIELD MARKS: _____

_____

FIELD NOTES: _____

_____

_____

_____

SKETCH PAD

DATE & TIME: _____

SPECIES NAME: _____

LOCATION: _____

WEATHER: _____

SIZE & SHAPE: _____

BEAK SHAPE: _____

WING SHAPE: _____

_____

COLOR/PLUMAGE: _____

FIELD MARKS: _____

_____

FIELD NOTES: _____

_____

_____

_____

SKETCH PAD

DATE & TIME: _____

SPECIES NAME: _____

LOCATION: _____

WEATHER: _____

SIZE & SHAPE: _____

BEAK SHAPE: _____

WING SHAPE: _____

_____

COLOR/PLUMAGE: _____

FIELD MARKS: _____

_____

FIELD NOTES: _____

_____

_____

_____

SKETCH PAD

DATE & TIME: _____

SPECIES NAME: _____

LOCATION: _____

WEATHER: _____

SIZE & SHAPE: _____

BEAK SHAPE: _____

WING SHAPE: _____

_____

COLOR/PLUMAGE: _____

FIELD MARKS: _____

_____

FIELD NOTES: _____

_____

_____

_____

SKETCH PAD

DATE & TIME: _____

SPECIES NAME: _____

LOCATION: _____

WEATHER: _____

SIZE & SHAPE: _____

BEAK SHAPE: _____

WING SHAPE: _____

_____

COLOR/PLUMAGE: _____

FIELD MARKS: _____

_____

FIELD NOTES: _____

_____

_____

_____

SKETCH PAD

DATE & TIME: _____

SPECIES NAME: _____

LOCATION: _____

WEATHER: _____

SIZE & SHAPE: _____

BEAK SHAPE: _____

WING SHAPE: _____

_____

COLOR/PLUMAGE: _____

FIELD MARKS: _____

_____

FIELD NOTES: _____

_____

_____

_____

SKETCH PAD

DATE & TIME: _____

SPECIES NAME: _____

LOCATION: _____

WEATHER: _____

SIZE & SHAPE: _____

BEAK SHAPE: _____

WING SHAPE: _____

_____

COLOR/PLUMAGE: _____

FIELD MARKS: _____

_____

FIELD NOTES: _____

_____

_____

_____

SKETCH PAD

DATE & TIME: _____

SPECIES NAME: _____

LOCATION: _____

WEATHER: _____

SIZE & SHAPE: _____

BEAK SHAPE: _____

WING SHAPE: _____

_____

COLOR/PLUMAGE: _____

FIELD MARKS: _____

_____

FIELD NOTES: _____

_____

_____

_____

SKETCH PAD

DATE & TIME: _____

SPECIES NAME: _____

LOCATION: _____

WEATHER: _____

SIZE & SHAPE: _____

BEAK SHAPE: _____

WING SHAPE: _____
_____

COLOR/PLUMAGE: _____

FIELD MARKS: _____
_____

FIELD NOTES: _____
_____
_____
_____

SKETCH PAD

DATE & TIME: _____

SPECIES NAME: _____

LOCATION: _____

WEATHER: _____

SIZE & SHAPE: _____

BEAK SHAPE: _____

WING SHAPE: _____

_____

COLOR/PLUMAGE: _____

FIELD MARKS: _____

_____

FIELD NOTES: _____

_____

_____

_____

SKETCH PAD

DATE & TIME: _____

SPECIES NAME: _____

LOCATION: _____

WEATHER: _____

SIZE & SHAPE: _____

BEAK SHAPE: _____

WING SHAPE: _____

_____

COLOR/PLUMAGE: _____

FIELD MARKS: _____

_____

FIELD NOTES: _____

_____

_____

_____

SKETCH PAD

DATE & TIME: _____

SPECIES NAME: _____

LOCATION: _____

WEATHER: _____

SIZE & SHAPE: _____

BEAK SHAPE: _____

WING SHAPE: _____

_____

COLOR/PLUMAGE: _____

FIELD MARKS: _____

_____

FIELD NOTES: _____

_____

_____

_____

SKETCH PAD

DATE & TIME: _____

SPECIES NAME: _____

LOCATION: _____

WEATHER: _____

SIZE & SHAPE: _____

BEAK SHAPE: _____

WING SHAPE: _____

_____

COLOR/PLUMAGE: _____

FIELD MARKS: _____

_____

FIELD NOTES: _____

_____

_____

_____

SKETCH PAD

DATE & TIME: _____

SPECIES NAME: _____

LOCATION: _____

WEATHER: _____

SIZE & SHAPE: _____

BEAK SHAPE: _____

WING SHAPE: _____

_____

COLOR/PLUMAGE: _____

FIELD MARKS: _____

_____

FIELD NOTES: _____

_____

_____

_____

SKETCH PAD

DATE & TIME: _____

SPECIES NAME: _____

LOCATION: _____

WEATHER: _____

SIZE & SHAPE: _____

BEAK SHAPE: _____

WING SHAPE: _____

_____

COLOR/PLUMAGE: _____

FIELD MARKS: _____

_____

FIELD NOTES: _____

_____

_____

_____

SKETCH PAD

DATE & TIME: _____

SPECIES NAME: _____

LOCATION: _____

WEATHER: _____

SIZE & SHAPE: _____

BEAK SHAPE: _____

WING SHAPE: _____

_____

COLOR/PLUMAGE: _____

FIELD MARKS: _____

_____

FIELD NOTES: _____

_____

_____

_____

SKETCH PAD

DATE & TIME: _____

SPECIES NAME: _____

LOCATION: _____

WEATHER: _____

SIZE & SHAPE: _____

BEAK SHAPE: _____

WING SHAPE: _____

_____

COLOR/PLUMAGE: _____

FIELD MARKS: _____

_____

FIELD NOTES: _____

_____

_____

_____

SKETCH PAD

DATE & TIME: _____

SPECIES NAME: _____

LOCATION: _____

WEATHER: _____

SIZE & SHAPE: _____

BEAK SHAPE: _____

WING SHAPE: _____

_____

COLOR/PLUMAGE: _____

FIELD MARKS: _____

_____

FIELD NOTES: _____

_____

_____

_____

SKETCH PAD

DATE & TIME: _____

SPECIES NAME: _____

LOCATION: _____

WEATHER: _____

SIZE & SHAPE: _____

BEAK SHAPE: _____

WING SHAPE: _____

_____

COLOR/PLUMAGE: _____

FIELD MARKS: _____

_____

FIELD NOTES: _____

_____

_____

_____

SKETCH PAD

DATE & TIME: _____

SPECIES NAME: _____

LOCATION: _____

WEATHER: _____

SIZE & SHAPE: _____

BEAK SHAPE: _____

WING SHAPE: _____

_____

COLOR/PLUMAGE: _____

FIELD MARKS: _____

_____

FIELD NOTES: _____

_____

_____

_____

SKETCH PAD

DATE & TIME: _____

SPECIES NAME: _____

LOCATION: _____

WEATHER: _____

SIZE & SHAPE: _____

BEAK SHAPE: _____

WING SHAPE: _____

_____

COLOR/PLUMAGE: _____

FIELD MARKS: _____

_____

FIELD NOTES: _____

_____

_____

_____

SKETCH PAD

DATE & TIME: _____

SPECIES NAME: _____

LOCATION: _____

WEATHER: _____

SIZE & SHAPE: _____

BEAK SHAPE: _____

WING SHAPE: _____

_____

COLOR/PLUMAGE: _____

FIELD MARKS: _____

_____

FIELD NOTES: _____

_____

_____

_____

SKETCH PAD

DATE & TIME: _____

SPECIES NAME: _____

LOCATION: _____

WEATHER: _____

SIZE & SHAPE: _____

BEAK SHAPE: _____

WING SHAPE: _____

_____

COLOR/PLUMAGE: _____

FIELD MARKS: _____

_____

FIELD NOTES: _____

_____

_____

_____

SKETCH PAD

DATE & TIME: _____

SPECIES NAME: _____

LOCATION: _____

WEATHER: _____

SIZE & SHAPE: _____

BEAK SHAPE: _____

WING SHAPE: _____

_____

COLOR/PLUMAGE: _____

FIELD MARKS: _____

_____

FIELD NOTES: _____

_____

_____

_____

SKETCH PAD

DATE & TIME: _____

SPECIES NAME: _____

LOCATION: _____

WEATHER: _____

SIZE & SHAPE: _____

BEAK SHAPE: _____

WING SHAPE: _____

_____

COLOR/PLUMAGE: _____

FIELD MARKS: _____

_____

FIELD NOTES: _____

_____

_____

_____

SKETCH PAD

DATE & TIME: _____

SPECIES NAME: _____

LOCATION: _____

WEATHER: _____

SIZE & SHAPE: _____

BEAK SHAPE: _____

WING SHAPE: _____

_____

COLOR/PLUMAGE: _____

FIELD MARKS: _____

_____

FIELD NOTES: _____

_____

_____

_____

SKETCH PAD

DATE & TIME: _____

SPECIES NAME: _____

LOCATION: _____

WEATHER: _____

SIZE & SHAPE: _____

BEAK SHAPE: _____

WING SHAPE: _____

_____

COLOR/PLUMAGE: _____

FIELD MARKS: _____

_____

FIELD NOTES: _____

_____

_____

_____

SKETCH PAD

DATE & TIME: _____

SPECIES NAME: _____

LOCATION: _____

WEATHER: _____

SIZE & SHAPE: _____

BEAK SHAPE: _____

WING SHAPE: _____

_____

COLOR/PLUMAGE: _____

FIELD MARKS: _____

_____

FIELD NOTES: _____

_____

_____

_____

SKETCH PAD

DATE & TIME: _____

SPECIES NAME: _____

LOCATION: _____

WEATHER: _____

SIZE & SHAPE: _____

BEAK SHAPE: _____

WING SHAPE: _____
_____

COLOR/PLUMAGE: _____

FIELD MARKS: _____
_____

FIELD NOTES: _____
_____
_____
_____

SKETCH PAD

DATE & TIME: _____

SPECIES NAME: _____

LOCATION: _____

WEATHER: _____

SIZE & SHAPE: _____

BEAK SHAPE: _____

WING SHAPE: _____

_____

COLOR/PLUMAGE: _____

FIELD MARKS: _____

_____

FIELD NOTES: _____

_____

_____

_____

SKETCH PAD

DATE & TIME: _____

SPECIES NAME: _____

LOCATION: _____

WEATHER: _____

SIZE & SHAPE: _____

BEAK SHAPE: _____

WING SHAPE: _____

_____

COLOR/PLUMAGE: _____

FIELD MARKS: _____

_____

FIELD NOTES: _____

_____

_____

_____

SKETCH PAD

DATE & TIME: _____

SPECIES NAME: _____

LOCATION: _____

WEATHER: _____

SIZE & SHAPE: _____

BEAK SHAPE: _____

WING SHAPE: _____

_____

COLOR/PLUMAGE: _____

FIELD MARKS: _____

_____

FIELD NOTES: _____

_____

_____

_____

SKETCH PAD

DATE & TIME: _____

SPECIES NAME: _____

LOCATION: _____

WEATHER: _____

SIZE & SHAPE: _____

BEAK SHAPE: _____

WING SHAPE: _____

_____

COLOR/PLUMAGE: _____

FIELD MARKS: _____

_____

FIELD NOTES: _____

_____

_____

_____

SKETCH PAD

DATE & TIME: _____

SPECIES NAME: _____

LOCATION: _____

WEATHER: _____

SIZE & SHAPE: _____

BEAK SHAPE: _____

WING SHAPE: _____

_____

COLOR/PLUMAGE: _____

FIELD MARKS: _____

_____

FIELD NOTES: _____

_____

_____

_____

SKETCH PAD

DATE & TIME: _____

SPECIES NAME: _____

LOCATION: _____

WEATHER: _____

SIZE & SHAPE: _____

BEAK SHAPE: _____

WING SHAPE: _____

_____

COLOR/PLUMAGE: _____

FIELD MARKS: _____

_____

FIELD NOTES: _____

_____

_____

_____

SKETCH PAD

DATE & TIME: _____

SPECIES NAME: _____

LOCATION: _____

WEATHER: _____

SIZE & SHAPE: _____

BEAK SHAPE: _____

WING SHAPE: _____
_____

COLOR/PLUMAGE: _____

FIELD MARKS: _____
_____

FIELD NOTES: _____
_____
_____
_____

SKETCH PAD

DATE & TIME: _____

SPECIES NAME: _____

LOCATION: _____

WEATHER: _____

SIZE & SHAPE: _____

BEAK SHAPE: _____

WING SHAPE: _____

_____

COLOR/PLUMAGE: _____

FIELD MARKS: _____

_____

FIELD NOTES: _____

_____

_____

_____

SKETCH PAD

DATE & TIME: _____

SPECIES NAME: _____

LOCATION: _____

WEATHER: _____

SIZE & SHAPE: _____

BEAK SHAPE: _____

WING SHAPE: _____

_____

COLOR/PLUMAGE: _____

FIELD MARKS: _____

_____

FIELD NOTES: _____

_____

_____

_____

SKETCH PAD

DATE & TIME: _____

SPECIES NAME: _____

LOCATION: _____

WEATHER: _____

SIZE & SHAPE: _____

BEAK SHAPE: _____

WING SHAPE: _____
_____

COLOR/PLUMAGE: _____

FIELD MARKS: _____
_____

FIELD NOTES: _____
_____
_____
_____

SKETCH PAD

DATE & TIME: _____

SPECIES NAME: _____

LOCATION: _____

WEATHER: _____

SIZE & SHAPE: _____

BEAK SHAPE: _____

WING SHAPE: _____

_____

COLOR/PLUMAGE: _____

FIELD MARKS: _____

_____

FIELD NOTES: _____

_____

_____

_____

SKETCH PAD

DATE & TIME: _____

SPECIES NAME: _____

LOCATION: _____

WEATHER: _____

SIZE & SHAPE: _____

BEAK SHAPE: _____

WING SHAPE: _____

_____

COLOR/PLUMAGE: _____

FIELD MARKS: _____

_____

FIELD NOTES: _____

_____

_____

_____

SKETCH PAD

DATE & TIME: _____

SPECIES NAME: _____

LOCATION: _____

WEATHER: _____

SIZE & SHAPE: _____

BEAK SHAPE: _____

WING SHAPE: _____

_____

COLOR/PLUMAGE: _____

FIELD MARKS: _____

_____

FIELD NOTES: _____

_____

_____

_____

SKETCH PAD

DATE & TIME: _____

SPECIES NAME: _____

LOCATION: _____

WEATHER: _____

SIZE & SHAPE: _____

BEAK SHAPE: _____

WING SHAPE: _____

_____

COLOR/PLUMAGE: _____

FIELD MARKS: _____

_____

FIELD NOTES: _____

_____

_____

_____

SKETCH PAD

DATE & TIME: _____

SPECIES NAME: _____

LOCATION: _____

WEATHER: _____

SIZE & SHAPE: _____

BEAK SHAPE: _____

WING SHAPE: _____

_____

COLOR/PLUMAGE: _____

FIELD MARKS: _____

_____

FIELD NOTES: _____

_____

_____

_____

SKETCH PAD

DATE & TIME: _____

SPECIES NAME: _____

LOCATION: _____

WEATHER: _____

SIZE & SHAPE: _____

BEAK SHAPE: _____

WING SHAPE: _____

_____

COLOR/PLUMAGE: _____

FIELD MARKS: _____

_____

FIELD NOTES: _____

_____

_____

_____

SKETCH PAD

DATE & TIME: _____

SPECIES NAME: _____

LOCATION: _____

WEATHER: _____

SIZE & SHAPE: _____

BEAK SHAPE: _____

WING SHAPE: _____

_____

COLOR/PLUMAGE: _____

FIELD MARKS: _____

_____

FIELD NOTES: _____

_____

_____

_____

SKETCH PAD

DATE & TIME: _____

SPECIES NAME: _____

LOCATION: _____

WEATHER: _____

SIZE & SHAPE: _____

BEAK SHAPE: _____

WING SHAPE: _____

_____

COLOR/PLUMAGE: _____

FIELD MARKS: _____

_____

FIELD NOTES: _____

_____

_____

_____

SKETCH PAD

DATE & TIME: _____

SPECIES NAME: _____

LOCATION: _____

WEATHER: _____

SIZE & SHAPE: _____

BEAK SHAPE: _____

WING SHAPE: _____
_____

COLOR/PLUMAGE: _____

FIELD MARKS: _____
_____

FIELD NOTES: _____
_____
_____
_____

SKETCH PAD

DATE & TIME: _____

SPECIES NAME: _____

LOCATION: _____

WEATHER: _____

SIZE & SHAPE: _____

BEAK SHAPE: _____

WING SHAPE: _____

_____

COLOR/PLUMAGE: _____

FIELD MARKS: _____

_____

FIELD NOTES: _____

_____

_____

_____

SKETCH PAD

DATE & TIME: _____

SPECIES NAME: _____

LOCATION: _____

WEATHER: _____

SIZE & SHAPE: _____

BEAK SHAPE: _____

WING SHAPE: _____

_____

COLOR/PLUMAGE: _____

FIELD MARKS: _____

_____

FIELD NOTES: _____

_____

_____

_____

SKETCH PAD

DATE & TIME: _____

SPECIES NAME: _____

LOCATION: _____

WEATHER: _____

SIZE & SHAPE: _____

BEAK SHAPE: _____

WING SHAPE: _____

_____

COLOR/PLUMAGE: _____

FIELD MARKS: _____

_____

FIELD NOTES: _____

_____

_____

_____

SKETCH PAD

DATE & TIME: _____

SPECIES NAME: _____

LOCATION: _____

WEATHER: _____

SIZE & SHAPE: _____

BEAK SHAPE: _____

WING SHAPE: _____

_____

COLOR/PLUMAGE: _____

FIELD MARKS: _____

_____

FIELD NOTES: _____

_____

_____

_____

SKETCH PAD

DATE & TIME: _____

SPECIES NAME: _____

LOCATION: _____

WEATHER: _____

SIZE & SHAPE: _____

BEAK SHAPE: _____

WING SHAPE: _____

_____

COLOR/PLUMAGE: _____

FIELD MARKS: _____

_____

FIELD NOTES: _____

_____

_____

_____

SKETCH PAD

DATE & TIME: _____

SPECIES NAME: _____

LOCATION: _____

WEATHER: _____

SIZE & SHAPE: _____

BEAK SHAPE: _____

WING SHAPE: _____

_____

COLOR/PLUMAGE: _____

FIELD MARKS: _____

_____

FIELD NOTES: _____

_____

_____

_____

SKETCH PAD

DATE & TIME: _____

SPECIES NAME: _____

LOCATION: _____

WEATHER: _____

SIZE & SHAPE: _____

BEAK SHAPE: _____

WING SHAPE: _____

_____

COLOR/PLUMAGE: _____

FIELD MARKS: _____

_____

FIELD NOTES: _____

_____

_____

_____

SKETCH PAD

DATE & TIME: _____

SPECIES NAME: _____

LOCATION: _____

WEATHER: _____

SIZE & SHAPE: _____

BEAK SHAPE: _____

WING SHAPE: _____

_____

COLOR/PLUMAGE: _____

FIELD MARKS: _____

_____

FIELD NOTES: _____

_____

_____

_____

SKETCH PAD

DATE & TIME: _____

SPECIES NAME: _____

LOCATION: _____

WEATHER: _____

SIZE & SHAPE: _____

BEAK SHAPE: _____

WING SHAPE: _____

_____

COLOR/PLUMAGE: _____

FIELD MARKS: _____

_____

FIELD NOTES: _____

_____

_____

_____

SKETCH PAD

DATE & TIME: _____

SPECIES NAME: _____

LOCATION: _____

WEATHER: _____

SIZE & SHAPE: _____

BEAK SHAPE: _____

WING SHAPE: _____

_____

COLOR/PLUMAGE: _____

FIELD MARKS: _____

_____

FIELD NOTES: _____

_____

_____

_____

SKETCH PAD

DATE & TIME: _____

SPECIES NAME: _____

LOCATION: _____

WEATHER: _____

SIZE & SHAPE: _____

BEAK SHAPE: _____

WING SHAPE: _____

_____

COLOR/PLUMAGE: _____

FIELD MARKS: _____

_____

FIELD NOTES: _____

_____

_____

_____

SKETCH PAD

DATE & TIME: _____

SPECIES NAME: _____

LOCATION: _____

WEATHER: _____

SIZE & SHAPE: _____

BEAK SHAPE: _____

WING SHAPE: _____

_____

COLOR/PLUMAGE: _____

FIELD MARKS: _____

_____

FIELD NOTES: _____

_____

_____

_____

SKETCH PAD

DATE & TIME: _____

SPECIES NAME: _____

LOCATION: _____

WEATHER: _____

SIZE & SHAPE: _____

BEAK SHAPE: _____

WING SHAPE: _____

_____

COLOR/PLUMAGE: _____

FIELD MARKS: _____

_____

FIELD NOTES: _____

_____

_____

_____

SKETCH PAD

DATE & TIME: _____

SPECIES NAME: _____

LOCATION: _____

WEATHER: _____

SIZE & SHAPE: _____

BEAK SHAPE: _____

WING SHAPE: _____

_____

COLOR/PLUMAGE: _____

FIELD MARKS: _____

_____

FIELD NOTES: _____

_____

_____

_____

SKETCH PAD

DATE & TIME: _____

SPECIES NAME: _____

LOCATION: _____

WEATHER: _____

SIZE & SHAPE: _____

BEAK SHAPE: _____

WING SHAPE: _____

_____

COLOR/PLUMAGE: _____

FIELD MARKS: _____

_____

FIELD NOTES: _____

_____

_____

_____

SKETCH PAD

DATE & TIME: _____

SPECIES NAME: _____

LOCATION: _____

WEATHER: _____

SIZE & SHAPE: _____

BEAK SHAPE: _____

WING SHAPE: _____

_____

COLOR/PLUMAGE: _____

FIELD MARKS: _____

_____

FIELD NOTES: _____

_____

_____

_____

SKETCH PAD

DATE & TIME: _____

SPECIES NAME: _____

LOCATION: _____

WEATHER: _____

SIZE & SHAPE: _____

BEAK SHAPE: _____

WING SHAPE: _____

_____

COLOR/PLUMAGE: _____

FIELD MARKS: _____

_____

FIELD NOTES: _____

_____

_____

_____

SKETCH PAD

DATE & TIME: _____

SPECIES NAME: _____

LOCATION: _____

WEATHER: _____

SIZE & SHAPE: _____

BEAK SHAPE: _____

WING SHAPE: _____

_____

COLOR/PLUMAGE: _____

FIELD MARKS: _____

_____

FIELD NOTES: _____

_____

_____

_____

SKETCH PAD

DATE & TIME: _____

SPECIES NAME: _____

LOCATION: _____

WEATHER: _____

SIZE & SHAPE: _____

BEAK SHAPE: _____

WING SHAPE: _____

_____

COLOR/PLUMAGE: _____

FIELD MARKS: _____

_____

FIELD NOTES: _____

_____

_____

_____

SKETCH PAD

DATE & TIME: _____

SPECIES NAME: _____

LOCATION: _____

WEATHER: _____

SIZE & SHAPE: _____

BEAK SHAPE: _____

WING SHAPE: _____

_____

COLOR/PLUMAGE: _____

FIELD MARKS: _____

_____

FIELD NOTES: _____

_____

_____

_____

SKETCH PAD

DATE & TIME: _____

SPECIES NAME: _____

LOCATION: _____

WEATHER: _____

SIZE & SHAPE: _____

BEAK SHAPE: _____

WING SHAPE: _____
_____

COLOR/PLUMAGE: _____

FIELD MARKS: _____
_____

FIELD NOTES: _____
_____
_____
_____

SKETCH PAD

DATE & TIME: _____

SPECIES NAME: _____

LOCATION: _____

WEATHER: _____

SIZE & SHAPE: _____

BEAK SHAPE: _____

WING SHAPE: _____

_____

COLOR/PLUMAGE: _____

FIELD MARKS: _____

_____

FIELD NOTES: _____

_____

_____

_____

SKETCH PAD

DATE & TIME: _____

SPECIES NAME: _____

LOCATION: _____

WEATHER: _____

SIZE & SHAPE: _____

BEAK SHAPE: _____

WING SHAPE: _____

_____

COLOR/PLUMAGE: _____

FIELD MARKS: _____

_____

FIELD NOTES: _____

_____

_____

_____

SKETCH PAD

DATE & TIME: _____

SPECIES NAME: _____

LOCATION: _____

WEATHER: _____

SIZE & SHAPE: _____

BEAK SHAPE: _____

WING SHAPE: _____

_____

COLOR/PLUMAGE: _____

FIELD MARKS: _____

_____

FIELD NOTES: _____

_____

_____

_____

SKETCH PAD

DATE & TIME: _____

SPECIES NAME: _____

LOCATION: _____

WEATHER: _____

SIZE & SHAPE: _____

BEAK SHAPE: _____

WING SHAPE: _____

_____

COLOR/PLUMAGE: _____

FIELD MARKS: _____

_____

FIELD NOTES: _____

_____

_____

_____

SKETCH PAD

DATE & TIME: _____

SPECIES NAME: _____

LOCATION: _____

WEATHER: _____

SIZE & SHAPE: _____

BEAK SHAPE: _____

WING SHAPE: _____

_____

COLOR/PLUMAGE: _____

FIELD MARKS: _____

_____

FIELD NOTES: _____

_____

_____

_____

SKETCH PAD

DATE & TIME: _____

SPECIES NAME: _____

LOCATION: _____

WEATHER: _____

SIZE & SHAPE: _____

BEAK SHAPE: _____

WING SHAPE: _____

_____

COLOR/PLUMAGE: _____

FIELD MARKS: _____

_____

FIELD NOTES: _____

_____

_____

_____

SKETCH PAD

DATE & TIME: _____

SPECIES NAME: _____

LOCATION: _____

WEATHER: _____

SIZE & SHAPE: _____

BEAK SHAPE: _____

WING SHAPE: _____

_____

COLOR/PLUMAGE: _____

FIELD MARKS: _____

_____

FIELD NOTES: _____

_____

_____

_____

SKETCH PAD

DATE & TIME: _____

SPECIES NAME: _____

LOCATION: _____

WEATHER: _____

SIZE & SHAPE: _____

BEAK SHAPE: _____

WING SHAPE: _____

_____

COLOR/PLUMAGE: _____

FIELD MARKS: _____

_____

FIELD NOTES: _____

_____

_____

_____

SKETCH PAD

DATE & TIME: _____

SPECIES NAME: _____

LOCATION: _____

WEATHER: _____

SIZE & SHAPE: _____

BEAK SHAPE: _____

WING SHAPE: _____

_____

COLOR/PLUMAGE: _____

FIELD MARKS: _____

_____

FIELD NOTES: _____

_____

_____

_____

SKETCH PAD

DATE & TIME: _____

SPECIES NAME: _____

LOCATION: _____

WEATHER: _____

SIZE & SHAPE: _____

BEAK SHAPE: _____

WING SHAPE: _____

_____

COLOR/PLUMAGE: _____

FIELD MARKS: _____

_____

FIELD NOTES: _____

_____

_____

_____

SKETCH PAD

DATE & TIME: _____

SPECIES NAME: _____

LOCATION: _____

WEATHER: _____

SIZE & SHAPE: _____

BEAK SHAPE: _____

WING SHAPE: _____

_____

COLOR/PLUMAGE: _____

FIELD MARKS: _____

_____

FIELD NOTES: _____

_____

_____

_____

SKETCH PAD

DATE & TIME: _____

SPECIES NAME: _____

LOCATION: _____

WEATHER: _____

SIZE & SHAPE: _____

BEAK SHAPE: _____

WING SHAPE: _____

_____

COLOR/PLUMAGE: _____

FIELD MARKS: _____

_____

FIELD NOTES: _____

_____

_____

_____

SKETCH PAD

DATE & TIME: _____

SPECIES NAME: _____

LOCATION: _____

WEATHER: _____

SIZE & SHAPE: _____

BEAK SHAPE: _____

WING SHAPE: _____

_____

COLOR/PLUMAGE: _____

FIELD MARKS: _____

_____

FIELD NOTES: _____

_____

_____

_____

SKETCH PAD

DATE & TIME: _____

SPECIES NAME: _____

LOCATION: _____

WEATHER: _____

SIZE & SHAPE: _____

BEAK SHAPE: _____

WING SHAPE: _____
_____

COLOR/PLUMAGE: _____

FIELD MARKS: _____
_____

FIELD NOTES: _____
_____
_____
_____

SKETCH PAD

DATE & TIME: _____

SPECIES NAME: _____

LOCATION: _____

WEATHER: _____

SIZE & SHAPE: _____

BEAK SHAPE: _____

WING SHAPE: _____

_____

COLOR/PLUMAGE: _____

FIELD MARKS: _____

_____

FIELD NOTES: _____

_____

_____

_____

SKETCH PAD

DATE & TIME: _____

SPECIES NAME: _____

LOCATION: _____

WEATHER: _____

SIZE & SHAPE: _____

BEAK SHAPE: _____

WING SHAPE: _____

_____

COLOR/PLUMAGE: _____

FIELD MARKS: _____

_____

FIELD NOTES: _____

_____

_____

_____

SKETCH PAD

DATE & TIME: _____

SPECIES NAME: _____

LOCATION: _____

WEATHER: _____

SIZE & SHAPE: _____

BEAK SHAPE: _____

WING SHAPE: _____

_____

COLOR/PLUMAGE: _____

FIELD MARKS: _____

_____

FIELD NOTES: _____

_____

_____

_____

SKETCH PAD

DATE & TIME: _____

SPECIES NAME: _____

LOCATION: _____

WEATHER: _____

SIZE & SHAPE: _____

BEAK SHAPE: _____

WING SHAPE: _____

_____

COLOR/PLUMAGE: _____

FIELD MARKS: _____

_____

FIELD NOTES: _____

_____

_____

_____

SKETCH PAD

DATE & TIME: _____

SPECIES NAME: _____

LOCATION: _____

WEATHER: _____

SIZE & SHAPE: _____

BEAK SHAPE: _____

WING SHAPE: _____

_____

COLOR/PLUMAGE: _____

FIELD MARKS: _____

_____

FIELD NOTES: _____

_____

_____

_____

SKETCH PAD

DATE & TIME: _____

SPECIES NAME: _____

LOCATION: _____

WEATHER: _____

SIZE & SHAPE: _____

BEAK SHAPE: _____

WING SHAPE: _____

_____

COLOR/PLUMAGE: _____

FIELD MARKS: _____

_____

FIELD NOTES: _____

_____

_____

_____

SKETCH PAD

DATE & TIME: _____

SPECIES NAME: _____

LOCATION: _____

WEATHER: _____

SIZE & SHAPE: _____

BEAK SHAPE: _____

WING SHAPE: _____

_____

COLOR/PLUMAGE: _____

FIELD MARKS: _____

_____

FIELD NOTES: _____

_____

_____

_____

SKETCH PAD

DATE & TIME: _____

SPECIES NAME: _____

LOCATION: _____

WEATHER: _____

SIZE & SHAPE: _____

BEAK SHAPE: _____

WING SHAPE: _____

_____

COLOR/PLUMAGE: _____

FIELD MARKS: _____

_____

FIELD NOTES: _____

_____

_____

_____

SKETCH PAD

DATE & TIME: _____

SPECIES NAME: _____

LOCATION: _____

WEATHER: _____

SIZE & SHAPE: _____

BEAK SHAPE: _____

WING SHAPE: _____

_____

COLOR/PLUMAGE: _____

FIELD MARKS: _____

_____

FIELD NOTES: _____

_____

_____

_____

SKETCH PAD

DATE & TIME: _____

SPECIES NAME: _____

LOCATION: _____

WEATHER: _____

SIZE & SHAPE: _____

BEAK SHAPE: _____

WING SHAPE: _____

_____

COLOR/PLUMAGE: _____

FIELD MARKS: _____

_____

FIELD NOTES: _____

_____

_____

_____

SKETCH PAD

DATE & TIME: _____

SPECIES NAME: _____

LOCATION: _____

WEATHER: _____

SIZE & SHAPE: _____

BEAK SHAPE: _____

WING SHAPE: _____

_____

COLOR/PLUMAGE: _____

FIELD MARKS: _____

_____

FIELD NOTES: _____

_____

_____

_____

SKETCH PAD

DATE & TIME: _____

SPECIES NAME: _____

LOCATION: _____

WEATHER: _____

SIZE & SHAPE: _____

BEAK SHAPE: _____

WING SHAPE: _____

_____

COLOR/PLUMAGE: _____

FIELD MARKS: _____

_____

FIELD NOTES: _____

_____

_____

_____

SKETCH PAD

DATE & TIME: _____

SPECIES NAME: _____

LOCATION: _____

WEATHER: _____

SIZE & SHAPE: _____

BEAK SHAPE: _____

WING SHAPE: _____

_____

COLOR/PLUMAGE: _____

FIELD MARKS: _____

_____

FIELD NOTES: _____

_____

_____

_____

SKETCH PAD

DATE & TIME: _____

SPECIES NAME: _____

LOCATION: _____

WEATHER: _____

SIZE & SHAPE: _____

BEAK SHAPE: _____

WING SHAPE: _____

_____

COLOR/PLUMAGE: _____

FIELD MARKS: _____

_____

FIELD NOTES: _____

_____

_____

_____

SKETCH PAD

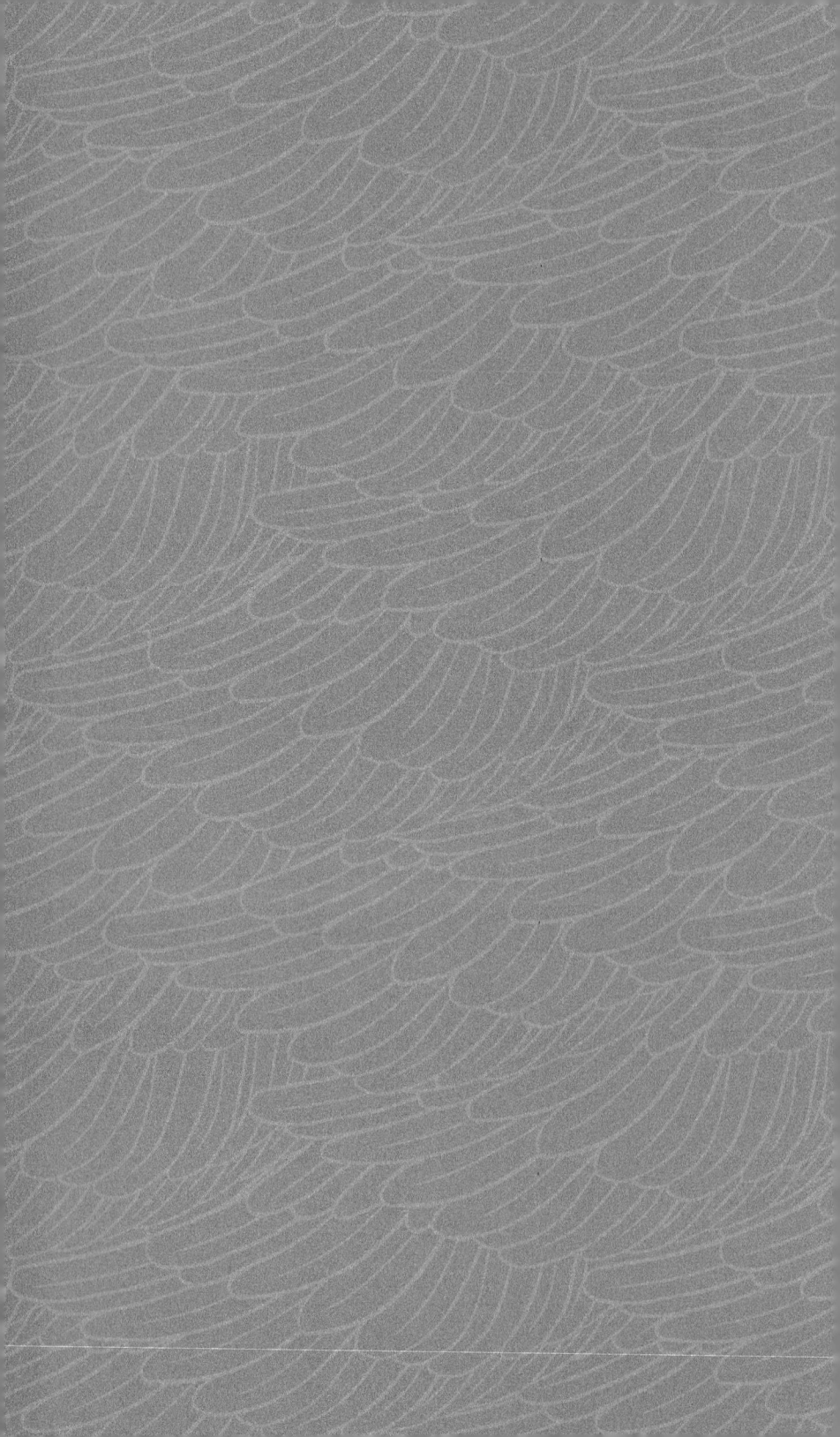

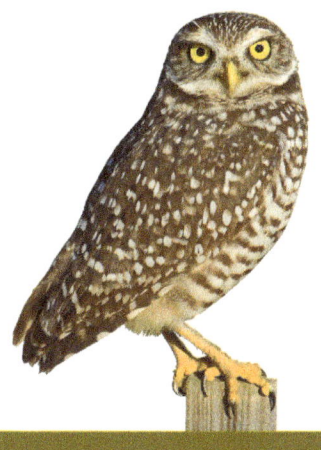

PART III

YOUR BIRD LIFE LIST

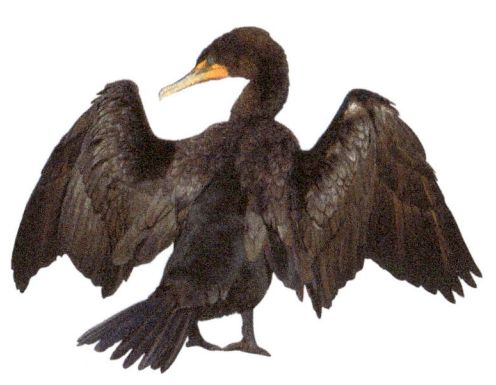

DATE	BIRD SPECIES	LOCATION

DATE	BIRD SPECIES	LOCATION

DATE	BIRD SPECIES	LOCATION

DATE	BIRD SPECIES	LOCATION

DATE	BIRD SPECIES	LOCATION

DATE	BIRD SPECIES	LOCATION

DATE	BIRD SPECIES	LOCATION

DATE	BIRD SPECIES	LOCATION

| DATE | BIRD SPECIES | LOCATION |

ABOUT THE AUTHOR

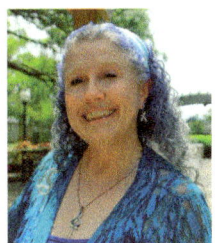

Kristine Rivers spent her childhood in a small Texas town enjoying nature and learning about birds and wildlife. As an adult, she loves sharing her passion with people of all ages, encouraging them to slow down and have fun as they observe the world around them. She founded Birding for Fun in 2015, through which she offers guided tours, workshops, and family-friendly events that embrace her philosophy that birding should be accessible to everyone. She is a proud Texas Master Naturalist and served as president of her local chapter from 2017 to 2019. She lives with her husband and several cats in that same small Texas town, where she creates driftwood art when not out exploring. You can find her at BirdingforFun.com.